Muscle Memory

Memory habits to strengthen your mind to be more productive.

Frank Knoll

Disclaimer

The author and publisher of this Book have used their best efforts in preparing it. The author and publisher make no representation or warranties with respect to the accuracy, applicability, or completeness of the contents of this resource.

The information contained in this Book is strictly for educational purposes. Therefore, if you wish to apply the ideas contained herein, you are taking full responsibility for your actions.

Trademarks mentioned in this book are property of their respective owners and may not be used without written permission. The fact that organizations, or websites are referred to in this work as examples does not mean that the author endorses the information, the company or website.

Readers should be aware that the information listed in this work may have changed or disappeared between when this book was written and when it is read.

Table of Contents

Introduction

This book has actionable information that will help you to increase your awareness effectively to get rid of stress and in an effort to be happy, and if you continue to practice your memory will get better. Other books that have helped with these processes are: The Power of Focus and the Ultimate Morning Rituals.

Imagine life without memories. Try to think of a life without any recollections of what has been. Without any idea of who you are, what you are and where you are. Just the simple idea of forgetting what happened after a night's drinking is terrifying. What more so if we don't have any memories at all?

This book is designed to help you understand memory. How it is formed and how do we lose it. This book will answer questions related to memory. What makes it possible to construct memories? Can you really trust your brain?

This book also outlines memory enhancing techniques to help you strengthen your memory. Which foods are best for the brain and which are not. And the effects of various things in relation to memory.

Read on, friend. And together, let us embark on a journey to make the most out of our mind.

Chapter I: Memory

Memory is defined as the innate ability to store, sort, process and retrieve information. Retention is also another name for Memory. It pertains to the concept of remembering things and experiences. Human memory is imperfect and has limited capacities. Long before, scientists believed that only one part of the brain is responsible for memory. Most experts are inclined to describe the brain as a filing cabinet wherein a memory is filed and stored. These experts say that when you want to recall something, you do it by accessing the file cabinets and sorting out through the files to get what you want to recall. But this idea of a filing cabinet is being greatly debunked nowadays. More researchers, through their studies, have found out that memory is in fact a much complex brain wide process. Different parts of the brain play a crucial role in the memory process.

"Humans, not places, make memories."
- Ama Ata Aidoo

Understanding the Human Brain
(Parts of the Brain and Memory)

To understand memory and the memory process, we must first understand the anatomy of the organ that enables the process possible. The human brain is a 3-pound organ that controls all bodily functions and interprets and stores information. In addition, the brain is also controls how we respond to certain situations. The brain is composed of three parts: the cerebellum, the cerebrum and the brain stem. The different parts of the brain control different functions. Damage to a specific area causes specific loss of function.

The Cerebrum is the largest part of the brain, which is subdivided between the left and the right hemispheres. It controls higher functions like touch, speech, reasoning, vision, hearing, emotions, and learning. The cortex refers to the folded appearance of the surface of the cerebrum. This allows for more surface area, which means it can accommodate more neurons. A single fold is called a gyrus and the groove between each gyrus is called a sulcus. Underneath the cortex are long connecting fibers called the axon. The cerebrum has distinct fissures which subdivided it into lobes. Each lobe serves a specific function. Despite the many subdivision of the cerebrum, it is best to understand that the lobes do not function alone.

- Occipital Lobe – this part is involved in the processing of visual information.

- Parietal Lobe – this part is located at the top of the head and processes sensory information.

- Frontal Lobe – the frontal lobe is involved in complex thinking. It is located behind your forehead.

  o Broca's Area – The Broca's Area is located in left frontal lobe. This part is responsible for speech production. Damage to this area may result to difficulty of moving muscles related to sound of production. The individual, however, may still be able to understand spoken language and read but will experience difficulty in writing and speaking.

- Temporal Lobe – the temporal lobe is located above the ears and processes auditory information.

  o Wernicke's area – The Wernicke's area is located on the left side of the temporal area. This part is responsible for speech comprehension. Damage to this area allows the individual to create speech sounds but is unable to interpret or understand. Individuals suffering from Wernicke's aphasia may speak in long and meaningless sentences.

The cerebellum and the cerebrum are connected by Corpus Callosum. This region is composed of bundles of fiber that serves as a way of connection between the areas. The Cerebellum is the part of the brain located almost at the base of the spine. The cerebellum is responsible for processing implicit memories. The cerebellum is also responsible for keeping you balanced.

The Brain stem is the part of the brain that includes the midbrains, the medulla and the pons. The brain stem acts as relay center that connects the cerebellum and the cerebrum to the spinal cord. This part is responsible for automatic functions like body temperature, circadian rhythm, heart rate, digestion, breathing, swallowing, sneezing, coughing and vomiting.

- Pons – this part of the brain stem that regulates relaxing and waking. This part is activated when you look at anything that is calm and relaxing.

- Reticular Formation – this part of the brain stem is involved in alertness and motivation.

- Medulla – this part of the brain stem regulates the automatic activity of the lungs and heart.

Neurons are the specific cells of the brain. It communicates which each other by sending electro chemical signals. Neurogenesis is the process of generating new neurons. This process is once believed to be impossible to occur in adults. Further studies reveal that, on the onset of new stimuli, even adult brains can create new neurons.

- Dendrites – branches of the neuron. A signal enters the neuron through the dendrites.

- Soma – this is the cell body

- Axon – cell extensions that send signals away from the cell body.

- Myelin Sheath – the myelin sheath protects the axon and speeds signal down

- Nodes of Ranvier – these are the spaces between myelin sheaths. Signals actually jump from nodes to nodes as they travel across the axon.

- Synaptic Vesicles – or Terminal Button are found at the end of the axon. These contain neurotransmitters.

- Synapse – this is the space between two neurons or between neurons and a muscle cell.

Deep structures

- Pituitary gland – this gland lies in a small bone enclosure located at the base of the skull. It is called the master gland because it controls other glands in the body.

- Pineal gland – this gland is responsible in regulating the body's internal clock and the circadian rhythm. The pineal gland can be found behind the third ventricle.

- Thalamus – this part is involved in the relaying of information from the body to the concerned part of the brain for processing. The thalamus plays a critical role in attention, pain sensation, memory and alertness.

- Basal ganglia – the basal ganglia is a group of nucleus that consist of the caudate, the globus pallidus and the putamen. The basal ganglia works together with the cerebellum to coordinate fine movements.

- Limbic system – this is the center of our learning, memory and emotions. This includes the hypothalamus, the cingulated gyri, the amygdala, and the hippocampus.

  o Hippocampus – the hippocampus is part of the brain responsible for transferring short-term memory to long term memory. This part of the brain takes charge of memories of shape and space. This part is also vital for declarative learning. Damage to the hippocampus hinders the formation of new long term memories. However, information stored prior to the damage is still accessible.

  o Amygdala – this is the part of the brain that regulates our fear response.

  o Hypothalamus – this part is directly involved in the regulation of the body's metabolic processes.

Neurotransmitters

Neurotransmitters are chemicals that allow transmission of signals between neurons.

- Acetylcholine – this neurotransmitter is the most abundant in the brain. It is involved in aiding your muscle to contract.

- Catecholamines – this neurotransmitter is involved in the reward-pleasure of the brain and learning. Types of catecholamines include epinephrine, norepinephrine and dopamine.

- Serotonin – this neurotransmitter can be found anywhere in the brain. It plays a critical role in the biological clock and emotional behaviors.

- Endorphins - this neurotransmitter is involved in hindering pain sensations.

"Memories, even your most precious ones, fade surprisingly quickly. But I don't go along with that. The memories I value most, I don't ever see them fading."
- Kazuo Ishiguro, Never Let Me Go

How Memory Works

Perception is the process of initial understanding brought by stimulation of any of our senses. As these stimuli comes into contact with our senses, our senses sends signals to the brain to process these information.

Memory Processes

1. Encoding – this is the process of transforming information into pieces which can be easily entered and retained in the memory network. There are two types of encoding: Automatic Encoding and Effortful Encoding.
   o Automatic Encoding – this is the unconscious encoding of memory chunks.
   o Effortful Encoding – this process of encoding information requires conscious effort and attention.

2. Storage – this is the process of retaining information pieces for future use.

3. Retrieval – this is the process of recovering information pieces back to the consciousness.

Human Memory Systems

- Sensory Memory Storage – serves as the holding storage for information, which are set for further processing and encoding. Iconic refers to visual information, which can be retained for about 3 seconds. Echoic refers to auditory information, which can be retained for only 2 seconds. At this stage, memory is very fragile and is prone to fading easily. Sensory memory is formed automatically without any interpretation or attention. To transfer information from the sensory storage to the short term memory, it needs to be properly attended.

- Short Term Memory or the Working Memory – processes information for long-term storage. Information on this storage is consciously and continuously worked on. Working memory declines with age. Interference and time can disrupt or alter memories, which are still being processed for storage. This is a limited and temporary storage of information. Pieces of information or chunks are stored for about 30 seconds to a minute. Without proper reinforcement, chunks stored in Short-term memory can be forgotten. STM can store about 7 chunks.

- Long Term Memory – This part encodes, decodes and organizes chunks for long term storage. Chunks in LTM can easily be recognized but not fully recalled since the information is still on the way to long term storage. Memories or information stored in the long term memory can persist for decades but is still not permanent. While reinforcement helps the brain to remember, a chunk of information needs to be associated or linked thoroughly to the brain's "network of information" to be properly retained in the long term memory. Long term Memory is subdivided into two different types of memory.

    o Implicit Memory (Non-declarative memory) – this type of memory involves memory without awareness. These are memory that can affect behavior however, it cannot be recalled consciously. Requires practice and rehearsal to be fully ingrained in the memory. Most implicit memories, once fully learned, functions on auto-pilot. Implicit memory are less likely to be forgotten.

        ▪ Procedural Memory – information that involves skills or the "how to". This memory allows us to perform things (like writing, reading or swimming) without much thought.

o Explicit Memory (Declarative Memory) – this involves memory with awareness or memories, which can be consciously recalled. It involves memory for concepts, facts and events. Explicit memory can be quite easy to acquire and to forget.

- Episodic Memory – this involves memories of significant events. It includes smells, emotions, sights, and sounds.

- Semantic Memory – this type of memory involves general facts or other information, which is not related to any personal events. It is associated with knowledge that we usually learn from school. It can include names, numbers, addresses and dates.

"Our memory is a more perfect world than the universe:
it gives back life to those who no longer exist."
– Guy de Maupassant

Stages of Memory

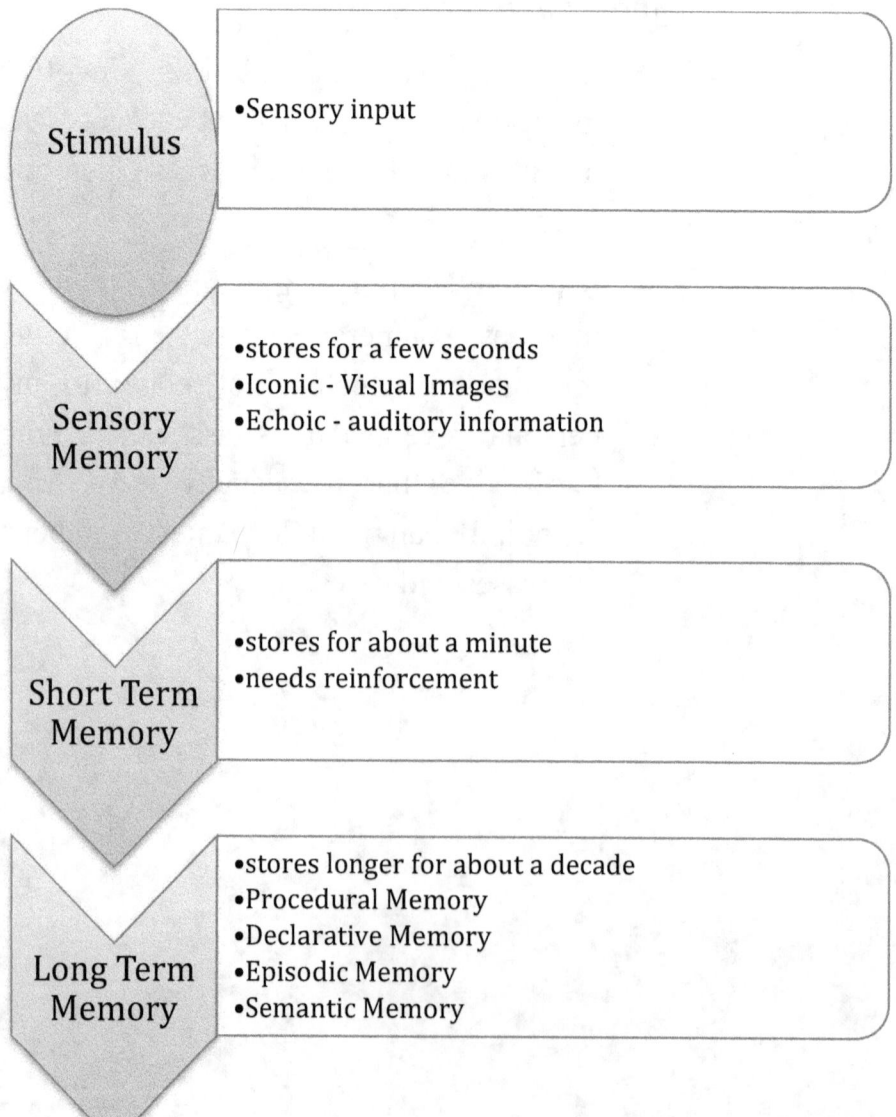

Stimulus
- Sensory input

Sensory Memory
- stores for a few seconds
- Iconic - Visual Images
- Echoic - auditory information

Short Term Memory
- stores for about a minute
- needs reinforcement

Long Term Memory
- stores longer for about a decade
- Procedural Memory
- Declarative Memory
- Episodic Memory
- Semantic Memory

Mind Deceptions

Constructed and False Memories

False memory syndrome occurs when one's identity or belief centers on strongly believed but false information. Experimental psychologists brought this phenomenon to awareness. Childhood abuse reported by therapy patients where speculated as false and therapy induced memories. A research study was then conducted to verify if certain memories can be created through similar therapy procedures. The research team chose a group of undergraduate students to participate in this study. Information about childhood events where provided by the subject's family members. The researchers then told the subjects that their family members provided four events about their childhood. Introduced via subtle hints, the researchers asked the subject if they recall the said events. One of the four childhood events is actually a false event created by the researcher, which the family members verified that the false event did not really happen to the subjects. The first group of students where asked if they remembered getting lost in the mall as a child and then being found and helped by an adult. The group of students believed that this event actually happened to them on three different occasions. In a related study with similar procedures, the subjects were made to believe that certain events happened to them when in fact, these events never really happened. The important thing to note here is that, whether manipulated through complex of simple methods, false memories are hard to discern from real memories.

Memory Distortion

There are times when memory is distorted as we try to assimilate in new information. Memory distortion can be done unconsciously. As we try to force in opposing and new information into our memory, our brain tries to distort our previous memory to accommodate the new one. Eyewitness testimonies are often unreliable because of memory distortion.

Misinformation Effect

Memory is reconstructed every time we recall it. This is the reason why memories are prone to distortion. The Misinformation Effect is a phenomenon wherein memory is distorted by the exposure of misleading information. This phenomenon is most evident during eyewitness testimonies. Eyewitness testimony is a crucial convicting evidence on any judicial court. But recent studies reveal the validity of these testimonies. Police interrogators pose misleading questions that ultimately distorts an eyewitness's recollection of the event. Furthermore, misinformation can happen even without intention to deceive. A group of eyewitness would often validate and contaminate each other's memories.

Optical Illusions

Our brain process information based on memory templates called schemas. This schema allows us to "see the whole picture" with just little clues. For example, if you heard the word "cafeteria", a memory template of a cafeteria will appear in your mind. Just by hearing or seeing the word "cafeteria", you'll instantly think about rows of tables, counters laden with food, an area for plates, trays and eating utensils, rowdy atmosphere, different aromas of food and the usual cafeteria noise. These descriptions are not necessarily true for every cafeteria but this is what a cafeteria would look like for you. These schemas are the reason why our brain deceives us through optical illusions. Whenever we are faced with images, our mind immediately makes assumptions of what we are seeing.

Ambiguous Illusions:

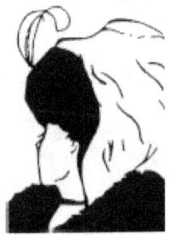

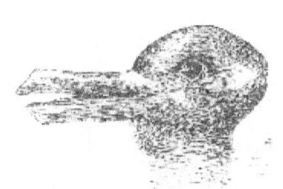

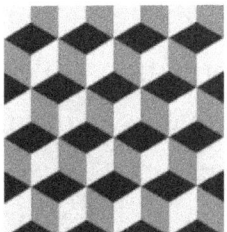

Is this a young woman or an old woman? (Look at the necklace until it becomes a mouth, or vice versa.)

Is this a rabbit or a duck? (Rabbit faces right, duck faces left.)

Are these cubes stacked right-side up, or hanging from above? (The black sqare can either be the top or bottom of the cube.)

"I can only note that the past is beautiful because one never realizes an emotion at the time. It expands later, and thus we don't have complete emotions about the present, only about the past."
– Virginia Woolf

Chapter II: Improving Memory

The Concept of Forgetting

Forgetting occurs when a chunk of information losses it's association or link to the brain's network. This is a natural phenomenon in the learning process. The first way Forgetting can happen is due to Encoding failure. This occurs during the sensory stage of memory. Disruption or interference, which can happen at any stage of memory encoding, processing and storing, can cause forgetting or formation of false memory. Memory is particularly vulnerable during the short-term memory. At this point, memory is most vulnerable to serial position effect. This is evident when in remembering a sequence, a part of the series overshadows another part. Proactive Interference happens when the first part of the series overshadows the rest of the series. This makes the rest of the series seem less important and thus less established. Retroactive Interference, on the other hand, occurs when the latter part of the series gets established better making the first part more prone to forgetting. For example, if you were given a list of names to remember, the principle of serial position effect suggests that most likely, the names in the top and bottom of the list will be remembered better. Interference also applies to prospective memory or the intentions of doing something in the future.

Amnesia is a medical condition that inhibits memory recall or retention which is possibly due to physical injury, illnesses or shock. It comes in two forms. Retrograde amnesia happens because of a physical trauma to the brain. This results in the disruption of short-term memory connection into the long-term memory. Anterograde amnesia, however, refers to the incapacity of the brain to form long-term memories. This can be a result of damage to the hippocampus or dementia.

Memories we no longer need are at a high risk of forgetting. Time is also critical in information decay. Passive decay is linked to the lack of purpose of a memory even at the encoding stage in the long-term memory. For example, contact numbers of your previous office will be forgotten since you no longer need to remember it.

Retrieval failure illustrates a situation where in recall of memory in the long term memory is difficult. One of the manifestations of this is the "tip of the tongue" phenomenon. You clearly remember the movie that you last watched, the story, the characters and even the actors who played in the movie, except the title of the movie.

Motives also play a role in remembering and forgetting. Repression is the unconscious forgetting of events or memories, which is possibly due to emotional trauma. The unbearable pain of reliving that memory unconsciously creates a mental block that prevents the brain from forgetting that memory. Repression is a defense mechanism of the brain to protect the body from severe emotional imbalance. Suppression is the conscious way of forgetting. To understand the distinction between repression and suppression, let us look at the case of identical twins Jake and Jade. Jake is physically abused by their father. Never a day goes by without a fresh bruise on Jake. Jade, on the other hand, as the favorite of their father is exempt from all the beatings. But Jade gets to watch his father beat his brother. Whenever his teachers ask Jake about his bruises, he always tells them that he did not remember how he got them. Up until Jake's accident, he insisted that he did not know how why he got bruises. The continuous abuse of Jake that ultimately leads to his death deeply traumatized Jade. Jade got hospitalized because of his extreme terrors. When he returned home, he no longer remembers having a twin brother. From this sample case, Jake is the one who suppressed his memories. Jade, on the other hand, due to the extreme emotional trauma of witnessing his brother being beaten to death, repressed his memory.

Why we forget.

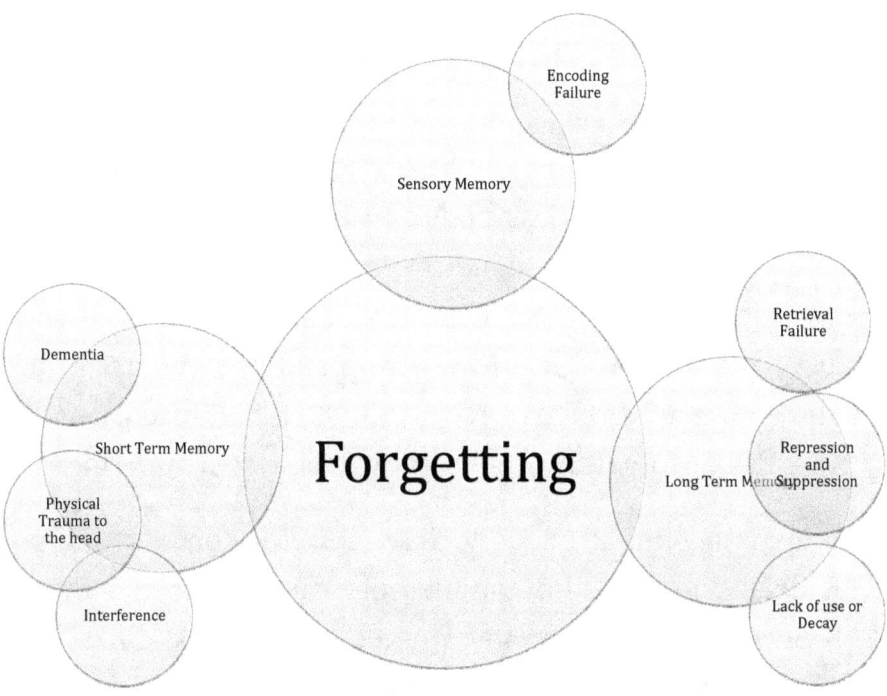

"Where does a thought go when it is forgotten?"

\- Sigmund Freud

The Mechanics of Remembering

Remembering is very crucial to our everyday lives. Imagine if your forget how to walk? How will you enter your house if you forgot your pass code? In case of emergency, how will you be able to contact your relatives if you can't remember their contact numbers? Have you ever thought about how it would feel to wake up and without any idea of who you are? Sounds creepy right? After discussing the concepts of forgetting, let us know tackle remembering.

A memory chunk needs to have several concrete links to be deeply ingrained in the memory. In the presence of new information, the brain immediately cross-links this information to the memory system. The more connection a memory chunk has, the least likely you will have to forget it. Cross-linking information also provides more clues that will aid in recall. There are several techniques to improve memory retention and recall.

Learning Styles

Although we all have the same brain structure, how we learn follows different ways. This is base on the premise of the Multiple Intelligence Theory. Howard Gardner popularized this theory in 1983. Gardner suggested that we have eight types of intelligence that corresponds to our individual talents and individuals. According to Gardner's

Theory, our strengths lie on identifying which type of intelligence we have. We learn better if we match our intelligence type to our learning style.

Retention and Measures of Retention

Retention can be measured in four ways.

- Relearning – Relearning involves recall of previously learned skill or information. It measures the amount of time needed to reach a certain level of competence. It can be used to measure either declarative or procedural retention. The time difference between learning and relearning is the important factor in this measure of retention. For example, a pianist learned the Flight of the Bumblebee when he was 5 years old. After 2 years, he was asked to perform the same song in a school recital. If it took him a month to learn the piece when he was 5 and a week of practice to perform it again after 2 years, we can say that the pianist has great retention.

- Reintegration – Reintegration involves the recall of complete memory from partial clues. This is commonly evident during essay writing exams and when answering puzzles.

- Recognition – involves the reproduction of the original content of the information, which the subject will identify as either true or false. Multiple choices and true or false exams are examples of this retention.

- Recall – this involves the repetition of previously learned information without giving any clues. This is evident through short item tests or fills in exams.

"We are all the pieces of what we remember. We hold in ourselves the hopes and fears of those who love us. As long as there is love and memory, there is no true loss."
– Cassandra Clare, City of Heavenly Fire (The Mortal Instruments, #6)

Factors that Affects Memory

Mnemonics

Mnemonics are remembering techniques used to recall information. This process involves encoding hard to remember information into an easier to remember ideas using visual images.

❖ Principles Underlying the Use of Mnemonics.
  • Association – method of linking together things, which need to be remembered.
  • Imagination – this is used to create and strengthen mnemonics
  • Location – this principle sets the boundary between mnemonics
❖ Types of Mnemonics
  • Method of Loci
  • Link Method
  • Chunking – process of breaking down information into a manageable unit for better retention. Chunking can increase the capacity of the short-term memory.

o Acronyms – information organization wherein a symbol is used to represent certain information. For example:
  1. 3BM(SHTR) – 3 Blind Mice (See How They Run)
  2. ROY G. BIV – Red Orange Yellow Green Blue Indigo Violet (colors of the rainbow)
  3. 26LOTA – 26 Letters Of The Alphabet

- Hierarchy – process of information organization wherein a complex idea is subdivided into categories and subcategories.

Memory and Sleep

Researchers suggest that the brain requires 7 to 8 hours of sleep a day to function efficiently. During sleep, the brain strengthens relevant information for better memory recall. Lack of sleep or little sleep can damage the brain's information processing, hinders long term memory and disrupts emotional stability.

Studies found out that sleeping after learning enhances retention of learning. This is because sleeping reduces interference. Listening to audio recordings before sleeping is said to have a positive effect on learning. We are able to remember most of what we hear before sleeping. This is due to the calm and relaxed state our brain enters before sleeping. A relaxed and calm mind is very conducive to learning.

Physical Exercise

The Brain is a Muscle that needs to be trained to achieve efficiency. Studies reveal that exercise contributes to overall heightened performance of the brain. Regular exercise can also lessen the risk of dementia. Athletic adults are shown to have better brain function than less active adult. This shows that even at old age, brain function can be improved just by engaging in regular exercises. Endurance exercises increase the concentration capacity of the brain. People became more attentive after undergoing rigorous exercise. Because the brain can concentrate better, information processing and retention is also more efficient. Physical exercise is also found to promote the release of hormones, growth factor and specific neurotransmitters. These specific neurotransmitters promote the learning process. In short, engaging in physical exercise not only makes you concentrate better, it is also signals the start of the learning process. And lastly, exercise has proven to promote the generation of new neuron cells. This process is called Neurogenesis. In a nut shell, exercise has the capacity to make you more focused, promotes the release of specific neurotransmitters and promotes the growth of new neurons. Studies also found out that listening to music while exercising increases verbal skills. Researchers suggest doing the following for optimal brain and body health.

- Resistance exercise at least twice to thrice per week.

- Stretching exercises involving major muscle groups at least twice daily. If your schedule won't permit the twice-daily stretching routine, try stretching before bedtime.

- Consider doing a daily aerobic exercise. For a vigorous exercise, 75 minutes a week of aerobic activity would suffice.

- Engage in Neuromotor exercise for 30 minutes a day, two to three days a week.

Stress and Memory

Studies found out that consistent exposure to stress results in a hyperactive amygdala and a smaller hippocampus. This is because of the elevated levels of cortisol, which is a secondary level of anti-stress hormones. Stress has been found out to promote brain aging and slows down the plasticity process. Stress not only promotes negative mood, it also decreases the attention focus of the brain. To keep your brain healthy, try to avoid stress as much as possible.

Social Relationships

Healthy social relationship is revealed to have an impact on the brain and cognition. Loneliness, for instance, is said to be a major factor in cognition decline among older adults. It also heightens risk of depression and dementia. Conversation allows for the exchange of information, which can be stimulating for the brain.

Video Games

Research shows that playing video games helps improve mental dexterity and boosts depth perception, hand-eye coordination, and pattern recognition. It can also improve information processing skills and attention spans. A study was conducted to verify the effects of playing games to the brain. Non-gaming volunteers are asked to play video games for a week. Researchers found an improvement in visual perception skills. Professionals who play video games are found to be more social and confident than their non-gaming peers. The popular notion that playing video games results in increased real world violence, however, is true. Consistent exposure to violence in video games can desensitize the brain, resulting to lesser response. This decrease in response does not necessarily result to violence.

Music

Listening to music activates the reward centers of the brain and reduces fear and other negative emotions. A widely popularized study claimed that listening to Mozart could boost cognitive performance. This results in a frantic effort of parents to help their children by buying Mozart CD's. However, this study is discrete when further studies revealed that the resulting cognitive boost is temporary and tiny. Nevertheless, Music training is found to actually increase the mass of the brain. Musicians possess bigger corpus callosum, motor cortex and cerebellum compared to non-musicians. No studies have proven that music training can make anyone smarter. It is proven, however, that music lessons can actually improve the spatial abilities of children. Music lessons can increase the reactivity of the brain stem to sound. The brain stem is involved in the basic encoding of auditory information. This can be further improved by continuous exposure to music.

"People have an annoying habit of remembering things they shouldn't."
- Christopher Paolini, Eragon (The Inheritance Cycle, #1)

Chapter III: Brain Training

Brain Gym

Try these proven techniques to help your brain stay fit and working.

1. Thinking Caps – this exercise aids in spelling efficiency, improves abstract thinking and listening activity and enhances the short-term memory.
   - Using your thumb and index finger, gently pull and unroll the top of the outer ear to the lobe. Gently pull the lobe and repeat three times.

2. Calf Pumps – this aids in concentration, comprehension, attention, endurance and imagination.
   - Stand straight and place your hands against the walls. Stretch your left leg behind you, making sure that your heel does not touch the floor and your body is at a 45-degree angle to the wall. Lean forward, bend your right knee, press your left heel on the floor and exhale. As you bend your knee, you will notice that your left calf is fully extended. Take a deep breath as you return from the starting position. Repeat for three times, alternating each leg. Remember to complete a breath with each cycle.

3. Cross Crawl – this exercise helps in reading, writing, listening and spelling, and it also enhances comprehension by coordinating the hemispheres of the brain.
   - Sit down and place your left hand across to your right knee as you raise it. Do the same with your right hand and left knee. Repeat for about 2 to 3 minutes.

4. Lazy 8's – this aid in the improvement of the visual attention and the mobility of the eye.
   - Visualize a point at eye level and align your body to it. The point will serve as the midpoint of the 8. Starting from the point and moving counterclockwise, move your finger up, over and then around. Repeat the steps, but this time, move your fingers clockwise. Repeat three times for each hand and then another set of three for both hands.

5. Brain Buttons – this exercise is capable of increasing blood flow to the brain.
   - Make a letter "L" with your index and thumb. Position it at the hollow spot below your collarbone. Lightly press this area in a pulsing manner. At the same time, place your other hand on top of your navel area and press. Press these points for about two minutes.

6. Energy Yawn – this simple exercise can relieve stress
   - Open your mouth as if to yawn and then massage the area where your jaws connect.

7. Positive Points – this exercise can help improve memory and relieve stress.
   - Lightly press with your fingertips the point above your eyes (halfway between your eyebrows and hairline). Close your eyes and inhale deeply and slowly for a few seconds. Release and then repeat two more times.

8. Hook Ups – this brain exercise lessens anxiety which is detrimental to memory
   - Cross your left leg over your right ankles. Cross your left wrist over your right and intertwine your fingers. Bend out your elbows and turn in your fingers so that it rests over the center of your chest. Take deep inhalations and exhalations while in this position for a couple of minutes.

9. Arm Activation – this exercise helps increase attention span.
   - Stretch your right arm above your head, extend your ribs. Support your elbow with your left hand. Move your arm forwards, backwards, away from your body and towards your body for a few seconds. Rest your right arm and allow it to hang comfortably at your side. Repeat for your left arm.

10. The Elephant – this exercise is suitable for children with attention deficit disorder as it activates all the areas of the brain.
    - Position your right ear over your right shoulder and extend your right arm to form the trunk of the

elephant. Relax your knees and try to draw the infinity sign on the ground with your right hand. Alternate arms after drawing a complete sign five times.

Proven Ways to Improve Memory

1. Choose which information you have to remember.
    - Studying does not require you to memorize whole books. Jotting down just the key points is enough to stimulate the brain.

2. Make the information meaningful.
    - When you read an article, try to grasp its overall context. Instead of memorizing the whole article, summarizing the article or laying out the key points will help you better to understand.

3. Make associations.
    - Our brain works like a spider's web wherein the insects are the information chunks. To keep the insects from flying, the spider bind them with more spider web. Likewise, if we fail to put in as much links to the new data as we can, we increase the risk of forgetting the new data.

4. Learn actively.
    - Involving the body actively while we learn is great way to retain information. Some people attest that pacing back and forth helps them remember more. Others incorporate dance steps while reviewing.

According to them, the dance step serves as a clue that aids in memory recall. This is especially true with individual who are kinesthetically intelligent.

5. Relax.
   - Nothing is more conducive to learning than a relaxed and calm mind. A relax mind can better recall any new information. So if you start feeling tired while studying, heed your body and take a power nap. You'll not only feel more refreshed and energized after waking up, you also be more capable of learning new information.

6. Create images and word pictures.
   - The part of the brain that processes verbal information is different from the part that processes visual information. By visualizing verbal information, you are strengthening the link of that information which is ideal for better recall. Try to create an image of a certain word. Mentally visualize the letters that comprises your chosen word. Think of other words that start or end with the same letter as your chosen word.

7. Repeat and recite
   - Verbally repeating information creates that same link as that of visualization. Saying things aloud activates the auditory sense when you hear it and the tactile sense of when you say it. Repetition is a popular remembering technique. Repeating things blazes the pathway through that certain information making it easier to recall.

8. Writing things down.
   - Repetitive writing works just like repetitive chanting would. Writing a note to remind you of something aids in recall even if you only see the note once. Most importantly, writing is a physical act that involves your hand, fingers and arms.

9. Tap your emotions.
   - Relating new information to emotions strengthens its link in our memory system. Your amygdala sends a chemical neurotransmitter that signals the brain to remember that information clearly.

10. Over learn.
   - To fight mental fuzziness, learn all you have to learn regarding a certain subject. This is like learning a skill. You have to practice until the new skill becomes second nature.

11. Go over the short-term memory rule.
   - Information in the short-term memory exist only for a minute. To go over the short-term memory rule, a quick review after each class could help you retain information better.

12. Study at the time of your peak energy.
   - Identify what hours you feel most energized. Studying during peak energy hours are shown to be more conducive to learning.

13. Distribute learning.
   - Try a short and spaced out study session instead of cramming the night before. Doing this gives your mind some time to relax and absorb the information as opposed to cramming everything.

14. Your attitude affects learning.
    - Information that opposes our opinion is more likely to be forgotten. Students who view math as difficult experience problem recalling mathematical equations.

15. Unleash your secret brain.
    - Try to avoid retroactive interference by allowing new information a time to settle in first before learning other things.

16. Create your own study technique.
    - All of the techniques listed here works best if you utilize them in combination. Try to develop your very own learning technique.

17. Take the long way to recall.
    - Whenever you experience "tip of the tongue" syndrome, try to recall everything linked to that information as much as possible. One way or another, you'll arrive at that lapsed information.

18. Notice when you remember.
    - Take note of the techniques that you use to remember things. This will help you adjust your learning styles to better suit your needs.

19. Use it constantly.
    - One cause of forgetting is lack of use. To counter this, access the information as much as possible.

20. Remind yourself to never forget.
    - Instead of saying that you don't remember, try to use a more positive self-talk. Say "I will remember" a couple of times to help you remember.

21.Mentally visualize a map.
- After visiting new places, mentally visualize a map of that new place. Do this every time you go to a new place.

22.Test your recall.
- Write down a list and memorize it. After an hour, try to recall as much items from the list as possible. Make the list as challenging as you can.

23.Solve math mentally.
- Try to solve as many math problems as you can mentally. Challenged yourself more by trying to walk while mentally solving math problems.

24.Challenge your taste buds.
- Do this exercise whenever you are eating. While eating, try to identify and name the different spices used in your food.

25.Join a cooking class.
- Learning to cook or finding a new way to cook can stimulate the brain. Cooking utilizes various senses, which activate different parts of the brain.

26.Learn a new language.
- The skills (listening and hearing) needed to learn a new language could stimulate the brain.

27.Refine your eye-hand ability.
- Learn new skills that enhance your fine motor skills.

28.Engage in a new sport.
- Engage in a physical activity that uses both the mind and the body.

29. Engage your senses.
    - Try to utilize two or more senses when you do something.
30. Listen to music.
    - Listening to music is actually beneficial for the brain.

Brain Training Apps – Lumosity

Lumosity is an application that offers scientifically proven brain enhancing games, which is suitable for all ages. It includes performance tracker so the player can monitor any improvements in his attention span, memory and creativity. Lumosity is created in the Lumos Lab as a cognitive enhancing tool for the Human Cognition Project. The project was collaborated with about a hundred leading clinician, researchers and teachers from various institutions around the globe. The Lumos Lab is a Research Company that specializes in neuroscience and brain training which is based in San Francisco, California.

Crossword Puzzles

A crossword puzzle is a square form word puzzle in grids of black and white. The main objective of the game is to fill in the white squares with letters that corresponds to the given clues. The white squares are numbered across and downward. The black shaded squares serve as spaces to separate words. Crossword puzzles became a popular addition to every newspapers and magazines worldwide.

Crossword puzzles are a great instrument to promote cooperative learning. Clues provided are divided between two groups: the Across group and the Down group. The Across clues corresponds to words that should be placed across the puzzle while the down corresponds to words that should be entered top to bottom.

Education

Across

1. Learner; one who studies
7. Opposite of *bottom*
8. Female deer
9. Preposition meaning "over and in contact with"
10. For example (Latin abbreviation)
12. And the others (Latin abbreviation)
14. Exclamation of surprise
15. Test; inspect closely
18. Not ever

Down

1. Tales; short fictional narratives; anecdotes
2. 2,000 pounds
3. Opposite of *down*
4. Rim; border; lip
5. Negative response; opposite of *yes*
6. Instructor
11. Conjunction used with comparative adjectives and adverbs
13. Vocal or musical sound; a particular pitch in an intonation
16. Objective case of the pronoun "I"
17. Roman numeral for *four*

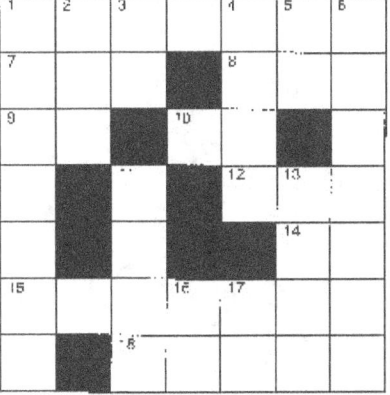

Sudoku and Kakuro Puzzles

The term Sudoku is an abbreviation of a Japanese phrase that means, "The digits must occur only once." This logic based number placement puzzle has been popular in Japan for some time and has already swept towards the United Kingdom. The goal of the game is to fill a 9X9 square grid with numbers from 1-9. The challenge of this puzzle is that each column, each row and each of the smaller 3x3 square grids should contain the numbers 1-9 only once. There are 9 smaller 3x3 grids in a single Sudoku puzzle. To start, each Sudoku puzzle contains seed numbers that serves as clues to find the solution. The Sudoku puzzle has only one solution.

6	5	9		1		2	8	
1				5			3	
2			8				1	
			1	3	5		7	
8			9					2
		3		7	8	6	4	
3		2			9			4
					1	8		
		8	7	6				

Kakuro or cross sums is also a popular Japanese Puzzle. This is a variation of the crossword puzzle. The goal is to find the numbers that when added, would be the same as the clues (sums) provided on top of each grid.

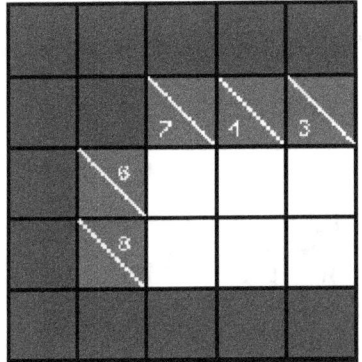 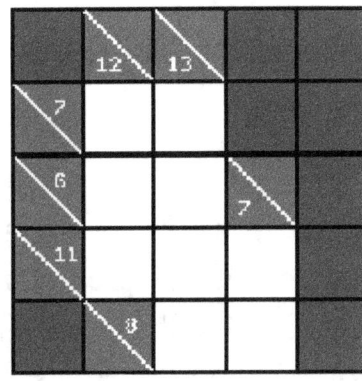

"If you wish to forget anything on the spot, make a note that this thing is to be remembered."
- Edgar Allan Poe

Chapter IV: Mindfulness Meditation

Mindfulness

Mindfulness is defined as a state of awareness or intelligence of the present moment. It is a fundamental practice in Buddhism meditation. It is a good way to promote memory functions and lessens the effect of stress. A study was conducted to glean the benefits of mindfulness on memory. For a month, subjects are supervised to perform 20-30 minutes of mindfulness meditation for 5 days a week. This study reveals that after a month, subjects exhibit a more positive mood and are less anxious, stressed or depressed. Subjects also reports improvement in attention and self-regulation. Brain analysis reveals that the mass of the gray and white matter in the brain increases along with an increase in the blood flow. Meditation is found to increase the density of the cerebral cortex, specifically those areas involved with sensation and attention. This is because of enlargement of blood vessels and the increase in number of support cells. It inhibits the activation of the amygdala and thereby prevents us from going on autopilot. The inhibited activation of the amygdala allows the areas of the brain related to learning, memory, psychological wellbeing and attention to be activated. This then results in enhanced learning capacity. It also clears up space in the memory network to enable new learning.

Mindfulness training is known to promote a positive sense of wellbeing and strengthens the attention capacity of the brain and the working memory. Regular mindfulness practice allows for better focus, concentration and attention. It also results in an enhanced intuition, confidence, self-belief and a greater ability to solve problem. Mindfulness exercises the brain muscles which then prevents memory loss.

Steps to Mindfulness Meditation

1. Close your eyes and do breathing exercises.
2. Focus your attention on your breathing.
3. After sometime, your attention will wander off your breaths. When this happens, shift your concentration back to breathing.
4. Think nothing except about your breaths.

Practice this meditation for about 3 minutes on your first try. Add two minutes after a week. Continuously add 2 more minutes as the week progresses.

"One of the keys to happiness is a bad memory."
– Rita Mae Brown

Chapter V: Brain Boosting Foods

Brain Foods

The foods that we eat affect our body greatly. This is especially true for the brain. There are certain food that greatly influences how our mind performs tasks, affects our mood and energy. Certain nutrients found in food can help enhance the different function of the brain. Below is a list of foods that when consumed daily can help boost our brain power.

1. Whole grain foods – whole grain foods contain high levels of Folate, which can then increase blood flow to the brain. A steady blood flow can do a lot of good for the body, especially for the brain. Whole grain foods also contain Vitamin B6 and Thiamine that can help improve memory. Half a cup of whole grain cereal or a slice of whole grain bread thrice a day could do wonders for not just for the brain but also for the heart.

2. Nuts – Nuts are scientifically proven to help clear the mind and enhance mood.
    o Walnuts – Walnuts are the most popular brain food. Physically, the walnut clearly resembles the human brain. The hard shell is the skull, the

thin sheet is the membrane and the walnut meat is like the brain's two hemispheres. Walnuts are rich in protein, omega 6 (linoleic acid) and omega 3 fatty acids (alpha linoleic acid), vitamin B6 folate, fiber and vitamin E; making it an excellent source of overall nourishment for the brain. Walnuts can also help control the serotonin level of the brain. Serotonin is a brain chemical that controls our appetites and moods. According to studies, Walnuts can help cure disorders commonly treated with antidepressants without exhibiting side effects. These disorders include depression, insomnia, compulsive behavior and overeating. Not only is this nut brain friendly, it is also good for the heart. Walnuts are also known to lower bad cholesterols in the body and can lower blood pressure.

o Cashews – Cashews are high in magnesium that can help open up the blood vessels in the brain allowing for more blood supply.

o Almonds – Almonds are rich in Phenylalanine which can help stimulate mood enhancing neurotransmitters like dopamine, noradrenaline and adrenaline. It is also rich in riboflavin that can help boost memory.

- Pecans – Pecans are a great source of choline. Choline helps in the proper brain and memory development.

3. Berries – berries contains antioxidants that helps the brain from suffering from cell aging.

- Blackberries – blackberries contain a nutrient called Anthocyanins. This nutrient helps protect our brain from oxidation stress and degenerative brain diseases. It is also known to reverse age related neurological deficits.

- Blueberries – Studies show that eating blueberries can literally strengthen the brain. It contains compounds that are known to activate the proteins in the brain to aid in memory and other cognitive skills. It can also increase the production of brain cells in the hippocampus. Blueberries are known to lessen the effects of age-induced conditions such as Alzheimer's disease and Dementia. It is also rich in Ellagic acid that can help prevent cell damage. Consuming at least a cup of blueberries a day can help protect the brain from oxidation stress.

- Strawberries – Strawberries are rich in antioxidants that can help improve the communication between molecules.

4. Seeds – just like many nuts, certain seeds can also help enhance the brain's power and boost positive mood.

- Pumpkin Seeds – Pumpkin seed is considered a Power food because of its high concentration of key nutrients. It contains Vitamin E and A, Omega 3 and 6 fatty acids and Zinc.

- Flaxseed –Flaxseeds can lower blood pressure levels in the body because of its abundant supply of omega 3 fatty acids (alpha-linoleic acid or ALA). ALA relaxes the blood vessels allowing for a better blood flow to the brain.

- Sunflower Seeds – Sunflower seeds are a great source of tryptophan. Tryptophan is a key amino acid that converts serotonin in the brain. In addition, Sunflower seeds are also rich in Vitamin B and Thiamine that are proven to help increase memory and other cognitive function.

5. Freshly Brewed Tea – Studies show that freshly brewed green tea can help strengthens the ability to focus, enhances memory, and fights mental fatigue. This is because of catechines that can simultaneously help the brain to relax and yet keep it focused. It is also proven to help boost dopamine that can create a positive mood state. Green tea is also rich in Polyphenols that provides a steady supply of glucose. Polyphenols can also help prevent heart attacks and cancers. Theanine, which is an amino acid abundant in any kind of tea, is known to activate the part of the brain related to attention span. At least three cups of tea a day would suffice to increase brainpower.

6. Eggs – For a 70 calories food, an egg is packed with various nutrients and vitamins. It is one of the best sources of high quality protein. It is also rich in choline that can help boost the brain's memory center. Choline

also has the capacity to double the size of the neuron which can help them fire signals stronger and rebound faster. Eggs are also great sources of two key antioxidants that lower the risk of age related eye problems like cataracts and macular degeneration. These antioxidants are called lutein and zeaxanthin.

7. Avocados – Avocados provide almost the same benefits as blueberries except for mono-unsaturated fats. This mono-unsaturated fat is essential in maintaining healthy blood flow through the brain. Consuming at least a quarter to a half cup of avocado proves to be very beneficial for the whole body.

8. Tomatoes – Tomatoes are rich in an antioxidant called Lycopene. This antioxidant helps protect cells against free radicals which are the main contributor to Dementia and Alzheimer's disease.3

9. Broccoli – Broccoli is another example of food categorized as a super food. It contains high levels of nutrient and is a primary source of vitamin K. This vitamin helps improve brainpower and enhances cognitive function.

10. Red Cabbage –Red cabbage is another great source of antioxidant polyphenols. Polyphenols helps lower the risk of brain cell damage and is important in preventing and treating Alzheimer's disease.

11. Eggplant – The skin of the Eggplant is rich in Nasunin, which is a nutrient that helps in enhancing the

communication between brain cells and messenger molecules.

12. Spinach – Researchers found out that spinach contain nutrients that can help protect the brain from oxidative stress and lowers brain function declines related to age. Accordingly, these studies found out that eating at least three servings of spinach (or other leafy vegetables like kale and collard greens) a day could lower age related brain decline by 40%. Leafy greens like spinach is rich in brain enhancing nutrients like flavonoids, carotenoids and folate.

13. Yogurt – Yogurt are rich in calcium that is proven to improve the nerve's function. It also contains tyrosine, which is a form of amino acid. Tyrosine is in charge of generating dopamine and noradrenalin that can enhance the brain's alertness and memory.

14. Chocolate –Chocolate, dark chocolate specifically, are known to be rich in powerful antioxidants and other natural stimulants which can increase endorphin productions. This results in an enhanced concentration and better focus. It also contains flavanols that helps in facilitating blood supply to the brain therefore enhancing cognitive skills. Milk chocolates, on the other hand, are known to enhance impulse control and reactivity and improve verbal and visual memory. Unfortunately, this super food is beneficial only if eaten in moderation.

15. Water – Water is essentially important on any part of the body. It helps the body metabolize hormones under stress. Water is also important in keeping neurons at a speedy firing pace.

16. Oily Fish – Wild salmon, Pollock or Cod are fishes rich in omega 3 fatty acids.

Nutrient base

These are just examples of brain food that we could indulge in to make our brain healthier. On a macroscopic level, the most important brain nutrients are:

- Omega 3 and Omega 6 Fatty acids – these healthy fats are essential for the brain because it helps protect the brain and aids in better functioning. Foods that are rich in healthy fats are oily fish like salmon, Pollock and cod. It is recommended to eat fish at least thrice a week. If eating fish is not applicable, fish oil supplements is your better alternative.

- Choline and Lecithin – Lecithin is the primary source of choline. Choline is the main building block of neurotransmitter that forms memory and thought. Foods that are rich in lecithin or choline are eggs, soybeans and wheat germs.

- Vitamins – essential vitamins such as Vitamin B, E, A, and K are related to better brain health and function. Leafy vegetables and colored fruits are main sources of these vitamins.

- Minerals – Minerals such as magnesium, calcium and potassium plays in important role in nerve function and helps in relaxing the brain especially when under stress. Nuts, Guacamole, banana, kiwi, grapefruit and potatoes are main sources of these minerals.

- Antioxidants – Antioxidants are substances that eat up free radicals to protect us. Free radicals are oxygen by products that damages other cells which results in aging and diseases.

- Fiber – Fibers regulates the steady stream of fuel for the whole body. Fibers are able to slow down the absorption of glucose for a more regulated fuel. Foods rich in fiber include vegetables, dried fruits, nuts, legumes, whole fruits and whole grains.

Foods to Avoid

Consequently, there are also foods that hinder or lessen the brain activity and functioning. These foods are better in moderation or avoided at best.

1. Simple sugars and syrups – Although the main consensus regarding the effects of sugar on the brain is varied, more evidence suggests that in small amounts, sugar can be beneficial in learning. However, a high level of sugar intake is found to interfere with memory functioning in the long run. For better brain function, it is best to avoid artificial sweeteners and limit natural sugars.

2. Saturated and Trans Fat – these unhealthy fats can increase the risk of bad cholesterol in the body. Saturated fats are found in poultry skin, full-fat dairy foods, meat and palm or coconut oil. These saturated fats also heightens the risk of intestinal and colon cancer. Trans fat or hydrogenated oils that are commonly used in commercial desserts and processed snacks. Trans fat are chemically produced from unsaturated fats and have no nutritional value. This also increases risk of colon cancer, cardiovascular diseases and even death.

3. Enriched, refined or bleached flour – This type of flour, whether bleached, enriched or refined, means that the flour is devoid of any nutrients. Using this flour increases risks of hypertension, diabetes, gum diseases, and obesity.

Stimulants

Stimulants are substances that directly affect the nervous system. This results in increased blood pressure, energy, heart rate, heightened alertness and breathing. Caffeine is the most widely known stimulant. Caffeine increases alertness and arousal by activating the central nervous system. Although in high doses, caffeine can cause anxiety, insomnia and jitters. A study revealed that two cups of coffee can boost the performance of the short term memory and the reaction time. Moreover, other researchers suggest that caffeine can protect older women against memory decline related to aging. Cocaine and amphetamines are also stimulants. These stimulants offer almost the same effects as caffeine although through a different way. Cocaine and amphetamines intake can increase the release of feel good neurotransmitter, like dopamine and serotonin, which results in high levels of euphoria. It is also known to increase energy and alertness. These results may seem positive but cocaine and amphetamines are highly addictive stimulants. In high doses, these stimulants can cause withdrawal syndrome and even psychosis. Severe withdrawal syndromes can lead to depression, which is the exact opposite of euphoria. That is beside the fact that an overdose of anything is fatal and dangerous.

Choline

Choline is an important macronutrient that plays a critical role in normal brain development, nerve and liver function, muscle movements, maintaining a healthy metabolism, and supporting energy levels. This water-soluble nutrient aids in methylation (forming of new methyl) which is important in the creation of DNA, in detoxification and in the transferring of signals between neurons. Choline also boosts brain function and aids in memory retention.

"I think it is all a matter of love; the more you love a memory the stronger and stranger it becomes."
– Vladimir Nabokov

Chapter VI: Training the Short Term and Long Term Memory

Improving Short Term Memory

1. Train your brain.
2. Utilize memory improvement techniques.
3. Consider memory-enhancing vitamins.

Improving Long Term Memory

1. Regular physical exercise.
2. Regular brain exercise.
3. Sleep well.
4. Avoid or reduce stress.
5. Eat a healthy and balanced diet.
6. Focus your attention.
7. Try mnemonic devices.
8. Replay new memories.

"There are memories that time does not erase... Forever does not make loss forgettable, only bearable."
- Cassandra Clare, City of Heavenly Fire (The Mortal Instruments, #6)

Chapter VII: Conclusion

All great things come to an end. This saying is true, even for this book. But the true purpose of this book would be forsaken if you don't take action. Everything in this book is doable. Every techniques and tricks practical. So there really is no reason to do nothing after reading this book. No matter how many books and researches you've read about the subject will be for nothing if you don't follow it. For without action, words are futile.

To strengthen your mind, you must do something. And I hope that this book will guide you towards the right actions and decisions.

"He was still too young to know that the heart's memory eliminates the bad and magnifies the good and that thanks to this artifice we manage to endure the burden of the past."
- Gabriel García Márquez, Love in the Time of Cholera

www.ingramcontent.com/pod-product-compliance
Lightning Source LLC
Chambersburg PA
CBHW071125280526
45787CB00003B/1170